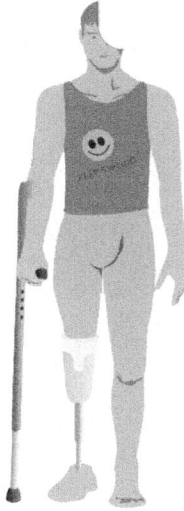

I Don't Want

My Leg
Cut Off!

Diabetic
Journal

Introduction

On April 16, 2016 I missed the bottom two steps because of the darkness in the stairs and fracture my fibula bone. Later that bone below the fracture was taken out. After now today, August 6, 2016 I have had 9 operations and close to $400,000 in bills. This was the last operation that I could have because the next one was below the knee amputation.

The problem was my blood sugar went wako(YES, new medical term) that the only way I can describe it. If you are trying to heal bones your blood sugar must be in the normal range. After the last operation I was in the nursing home and was given insulin shots at all my meals and in the morning.

Here I went to pricking my fingers to draw blood to test blood sugar. I have a device in which I can record my blood sugar on my iPhone. It is DARIO. My doctor loves it because it can show him at a quick glance what is going on in my daily schedule. (I do not get any commission for mention this product.)

Everyday I am improving my blood sugar scores and taking my insulin. I have change my diet and exercise which is hard at this time because I am unable to walk because of the surgery on the left foot.

Bless you on your JOURNEY, GARY

Name _____

Doctor's Name

_____

Doctor's phone number

_____

Hospital phone number

_____

Family member to contact

_____

Pharmacy

_____

Medication for Insulin:
_____

Date		AM	NOON	SUPPER	BEDTIME	WEIGHT
	Sugar					
	Insulin					
	Sugar					
	Insulin					
	Sugar					
	Insulin					
	Sugar					
	Insulin					
	Sugar					
	Insulin					
	Sugar					
	Insulin					
	Sugar					
	Insulin					

Long Term Insulin usually in the morning—Check with Doctor.   Short term Insulin taken with the meals—Check with Doctor.   He will give you instruction looking like this.

Accucheck of 100—150= 2 units. 151-200=4 units. 201—250=6 units. 251-300=8 units.301-350=10 units. 351-400=12 units.

(CHECK WITH YOUR DOCTOR ON YOUR OWN INSULIN TO BE ADDED TO THE BASE UNIT. MY BASE UNIT WAS 10, IF MY SUGAR WAS 125 THAT WOULD 2+10=12 UNITS THAT MORNING.)

— Long Term Insulin usually in the morning Check with Doctor.

Short term Insulin taken with the meals—Check with Doctor.

He will give you instruction looking like this.

Accucheck of 100—150= 2 units.

151-200=4 units. 201—250=6 units. 251-300=8 units.   301-350=10 units. 351-400=12 units.

(CHECK WITH YOUR DOCTOR ON YOUR OWN INSULIN TO BE ADDED TO THE BASE UNIT. My base unit was 10, if my sugar was 125 that would be 2+10=12 units for that morning.)

My Accucheck from my Doctor:

(Write it below each level and insulin)

Weekly Plans

Sunday

Monday

Tuesday

Wednesday

Thursday

Friday

Saturday

What you could do with the Weekly Plan page?

You could write what you ate for the day.

You could write when you exercise and how long.

You could make a grocery list if you needed to in order to get healthy.

Weekly Plans

	Sunday

	Monday

	Tuesday

	Wednesday

	Thursday

	Friday

	Saturday

Date		AM	NOON	SUPPER	BEDTIME	WEIGHT
	Sugar					
	Insulin					
	Sugar					
	Insulin					
	Sugar					
	Insulin					
	Sugar					
	Insulin					
	Sugar					
	Insulin					
	Sugar					
	Insulin					
	Sugar					
	Insulin					

Weekly Meal Plan

Breakfast	Lunch	Dinner	Snacks	
				Sunday

Breakfast	Lunch	Dinner	Snacks	
				Monday

Breakfast	Lunch	Dinner	Snacks	
				Tuesday

Breakfast	Lunch	Dinner	Snacks	
				Wednesday

Breakfast	Lunch	Dinner	Snacks	
				Thursday

Breakfast	Lunch	Dinner	Snacks	
				Friday

Breakfast	Lunch	Dinner	Snacks	
				Saturday

Notes:

Food & Fitness Tracker

WEEK: _____

STARTING WEIGHT: _____

	CALORIE INTAKE		EXERCISE		
MON	BRKFST:		TYPE	TIME	CAL. BURNED
	LUNCH:				
	DINNER:				
	SNACKS:	BEVERAGES:			
	TOTAL CALORIE INTAKE:		**TOTAL CALORIES BURNED:**		
TUE	BRKFST:		TYPE	TIME	CAL. BURNED
	LUNCH:				
	DINNER:				
	SNACKS:	BEVERAGES:			
	TOTAL CALORIE INTAKE:		**TOTAL CALORIES BURNED:**		
WED	BRKFST:		TYPE	TIME	CAL. BURNED
	LUNCH:				
	DINNER:				
	SNACKS:	BEVERAGES:			
	TOTAL CALORIE INTAKE:		**TOTAL CALORIES BURNED:**		
THU	BRKFST:		TYPE	TIME	CAL. BURNED
	LUNCH:				
	DINNER:				
	SNACKS:	BEVERAGES:			
	TOTAL CALORIE INTAKE:		**TOTAL CALORIES BURNED:**		
FRI	BRKFST:		TYPE	TIME	CAL. BURNED
	LUNCH:				
	DINNER:				
	SNACKS:	BEVERAGES:			
	TOTAL CALORIE INTAKE:		**TOTAL CALORIES BURNED:**		
SAT	BRKFST:		TYPE	TIME	CAL. BURNED
	LUNCH:				
	DINNER:				
	SNACKS:	BEVERAGES:			
	TOTAL CALORIE INTAKE:		**TOTAL CALORIES BURNED:**		
SUN	BRKFST:		TYPE	TIME	CAL. BURNED
	LUNCH:				
	DINNER:				
	SNACKS:	BEVERAGES:			

ENDING WEIGHT: _____   Lost/Gained _____

Weekly Plans

Sunday

Monday

Tuesday

Wednesday

Thursday

Friday

Saturday

Date		AM	NOON	SUPPER	BEDTIME	WEIGHT
	Sugar					
	Insulin					
	Sugar					
	Insulin					
	Sugar					
	Insulin					
	Sugar					
	Insulin					
	Sugar					
	Insulin					
	Sugar					
	Insulin					
	Sugar					
	Insulin					

Weekly Meal Plan

Breakfast	Lunch	Dinner	Snacks	Sunday

Breakfast	Lunch	Dinner	Snacks	Monday

Breakfast	Lunch	Dinner	Snacks	Tuesday

Breakfast	Lunch	Dinner	Snacks	Wednesday

Breakfast	Lunch	Dinner	Snacks	Thursday

Breakfast	Lunch	Dinner	Snacks	Friday

Breakfast	Lunch	Dinner	Snacks	Saturday

Notes:

Food & Fitness Tracker

WEEK: _____

STARTING WEIGHT: _____

	CALORIE INTAKE		EXERCISE		
MON	BRKFST:		TYPE	TIME	CAL. BURNED
	LUNCH:				
	DINNER:				
	SNACKS:	BEVERAGES:			
	TOTAL CALORIE INTAKE:		TOTAL CALORIES BURNED:		
TUE	BRKFST:		TYPE	TIME	CAL. BURNED
	LUNCH:				
	DINNER:				
	SNACKS:	BEVERAGES:			
	TOTAL CALORIE INTAKE:		TOTAL CALORIES BURNED:		
WED	BRKFST:		TYPE	TIME	CAL. BURNED
	LUNCH:				
	DINNER:				
	SNACKS:	BEVERAGES:			
	TOTAL CALORIE INTAKE:		TOTAL CALORIES BURNED:		
THU	BRKFST:		TYPE	TIME	CAL. BURNED
	LUNCH:				
	DINNER:				
	SNACKS:	BEVERAGES:			
	TOTAL CALORIE INTAKE:		TOTAL CALORIES BURNED:		
FRI	BRKFST:		TYPE	TIME	CAL. BURNED
	LUNCH:				
	DINNER:				
	SNACKS:	BEVERAGES:			
	TOTAL CALORIE INTAKE:		TOTAL CALORIES BURNED:		
SAT	BRKFST:		TYPE	TIME	CAL. BURNED
	LUNCH:				
	DINNER:				
	SNACKS:	BEVERAGES:			
	TOTAL CALORIE INTAKE:		TOTAL CALORIES BURNED:		
SUN	BRKFST:		TYPE	TIME	CAL. BURNED
	LUNCH:				
	DINNER:				
	SNACKS:	BEVERAGES:			

ENDING WEIGHT: _____   Lost/Gained _____

Weekly Meal Plan

Breakfast	Lunch	Dinner	Snacks	
				Sunday

Breakfast	Lunch	Dinner	Snacks	
				Monday

Breakfast	Lunch	Dinner	Snacks	
				Tuesday

Breakfast	Lunch	Dinner	Snacks	
				Wednesday

Breakfast	Lunch	Dinner	Snacks	
				Thursday

Breakfast	Lunch	Dinner	Snacks	
				Friday

Breakfast	Lunch	Dinner	Snacks	
				Saturday

Notes:

Food & Fitness Tracker

WEEK:_____

STARTING WEIGHT: _____

	CALORIE INTAKE		EXERCISE		
MON	BRKFST:		TYPE	TIME	CAL. BURNED
	LUNCH:				
	DINNER:				
	SNACKS:	BEVERAGES:			
	TOTAL CALORIE INTAKE:		TOTAL CALORIES BURNED:		
TUE	BRKFST:		TYPE	TIME	CAL. BURNED
	LUNCH:				
	DINNER:				
	SNACKS:	BEVERAGES:			
	TOTAL CALORIE INTAKE:		TOTAL CALORIES BURNED:		
WED	BRKFST:		TYPE	TIME	CAL. BURNED
	LUNCH:				
	DINNER:				
	SNACKS:	BEVERAGES:			
	TOTAL CALORIE INTAKE:		TOTAL CALORIES BURNED:		
THU	BRKFST:		TYPE	TIME	CAL. BURNED
	LUNCH:				
	DINNER:				
	SNACKS:	BEVERAGES:			
	TOTAL CALORIE INTAKE:		TOTAL CALORIES BURNED:		
FRI	BRKFST:		TYPE	TIME	CAL. BURNED
	LUNCH:				
	DINNER:				
	SNACKS:	BEVERAGES:			
	TOTAL CALORIE INTAKE:		TOTAL CALORIES BURNED:		
SAT	BRKFST:		TYPE	TIME	CAL. BURNED
	LUNCH:				
	DINNER:				
	SNACKS:	BEVERAGES:			
	TOTAL CALORIE INTAKE:		TOTAL CALORIES BURNED:		
SUN	BRKFST:		TYPE	TIME	CAL. BURNED
	LUNCH:				
	DINNER:				
	SNACKS:	BEVERAGES:			

ENDING WEIGHT: _____   Lost/Gained _____

Weekly Plans

Sunday

Monday

Tuesday

Wednesday

Thursday

Friday

Saturday

Date		AM	NOON	SUPPER	BEDTIME	WEIGHT
	Sugar					
	Insulin					
	Sugar					
	Insulin					
	Sugar					
	Insulin					
	Sugar					
	Insulin					
	Sugar					
	Insulin					
	Sugar					
	Insulin					
	Sugar					
	Insulin					

Weekly Meal Plan

Breakfast	Lunch	Dinner	Snacks	Sunday

Breakfast	Lunch	Dinner	Snacks	Monday

Breakfast	Lunch	Dinner	Snacks	Tuesday

Breakfast	Lunch	Dinner	Snacks	Wednesday

Breakfast	Lunch	Dinner	Snacks	Thursday

Breakfast	Lunch	Dinner	Snacks	Friday

Breakfast	Lunch	Dinner	Snacks	Saturday

Notes:

Food & Fitness Tracker

WEEK: _____

STARTING WEIGHT: _____

	CALORIE INTAKE		EXERCISE		
MON	BRKFST:		TYPE	TIME	CAL. BURNED
	LUNCH:				
	DINNER:				
	SNACKS:	BEVERAGES:			
	TOTAL CALORIE INTAKE:		**TOTAL CALORIES BURNED:**		
TUE	BRKFST:		TYPE	TIME	CAL. BURNED
	LUNCH:				
	DINNER:				
	SNACKS:	BEVERAGES:			
	TOTAL CALORIE INTAKE:		**TOTAL CALORIES BURNED:**		
WED	BRKFST:		TYPE	TIME	CAL. BURNED
	LUNCH:				
	DINNER:				
	SNACKS:	BEVERAGES:			
	TOTAL CALORIE INTAKE:		**TOTAL CALORIES BURNED:**		
THU	BRKFST:		TYPE	TIME	CAL. BURNED
	LUNCH:				
	DINNER:				
	SNACKS:	BEVERAGES:			
	TOTAL CALORIE INTAKE:		**TOTAL CALORIES BURNED:**		
FRI	BRKFST:		TYPE	TIME	CAL. BURNED
	LUNCH:				
	DINNER:				
	SNACKS:	BEVERAGES:			
	TOTAL CALORIE INTAKE:		**TOTAL CALORIES BURNED:**		
SAT	BRKFST:		TYPE	TIME	CAL. BURNED
	LUNCH:				
	DINNER:				
	SNACKS:	BEVERAGES:			
	TOTAL CALORIE INTAKE:		**TOTAL CALORIES BURNED:**		
SUN	BRKFST:		TYPE	TIME	CAL. BURNED
	LUNCH:				
	DINNER:				
	SNACKS:	BEVERAGES:			

ENDING WEIGHT: _____   Lost/Gained _____

Weekly Plans

	Sunday
	Monday
	Tuesday
	Wednesday
	Thursday
	Friday
	Saturday

Date		AM	NOON	SUPPER	BEDTIME	WEIGHT
	Sugar					
	Insulin					
	Sugar					
	Insulin					
	Sugar					
	Insulin					
	Sugar					
	Insulin					
	Sugar					
	Insulin					
	Sugar					
	Insulin					
	Sugar					
	Insulin					

Weekly Meal Plan

Breakfast	Lunch	Dinner	Snacks	Sunday
Breakfast	Lunch	Dinner	Snacks	Monday
Breakfast	Lunch	Dinner	Snacks	Tuesday
Breakfast	Lunch	Dinner	Snacks	Wednesday
Breakfast	Lunch	Dinner	Snacks	Thursday
Breakfast	Lunch	Dinner	Snacks	Friday
Breakfast	Lunch	Dinner	Snacks	Saturday

Notes:

Food & Fitness Tracker

WEEK: _____

STARTING WEIGHT: _____

	CALORIE INTAKE		EXERCISE		
MON	BRKFST:		TYPE	TIME	CAL. BURNED
	LUNCH:				
	DINNER:				
	SNACKS:	BEVERAGES:			
	TOTAL CALORIE INTAKE:		TOTAL CALORIES BURNED:		
TUE	BRKFST:		TYPE	TIME	CAL. BURNED
	LUNCH:				
	DINNER:				
	SNACKS:	BEVERAGES:			
	TOTAL CALORIE INTAKE:		TOTAL CALORIES BURNED:		
WED	BRKFST:		TYPE	TIME	CAL. BURNED
	LUNCH:				
	DINNER:				
	SNACKS:	BEVERAGES:			
	TOTAL CALORIE INTAKE:		TOTAL CALORIES BURNED:		
THU	BRKFST:		TYPE	TIME	CAL. BURNED
	LUNCH:				
	DINNER:				
	SNACKS:	BEVERAGES:			
	TOTAL CALORIE INTAKE:		TOTAL CALORIES BURNED:		
FRI	BRKFST:		TYPE	TIME	CAL. BURNED
	LUNCH:				
	DINNER:				
	SNACKS:	BEVERAGES:			
	TOTAL CALORIE INTAKE:		TOTAL CALORIES BURNED:		
SAT	BRKFST:		TYPE	TIME	CAL. BURNED
	LUNCH:				
	DINNER:				
	SNACKS:	BEVERAGES:			
	TOTAL CALORIE INTAKE:		TOTAL CALORIES BURNED:		
SUN	BRKFST:		TYPE	TIME	CAL. BURNED
	LUNCH:				
	DINNER:				
	SNACKS:	BEVERAGES:			

ENDING WEIGHT: _____

Lost/Gained _____

Weekly Plans

	Sunday

	Monday

	Tuesday

	Wednesday

	Thursday

	Friday

	Saturday

Date		AM	NOON	SUPPER	BEDTIME	WEIGHT
	Sugar					
	Insulin					
	Sugar					
	Insulin					
	Sugar					
	Insulin					
	Sugar					
	Insulin					
	Sugar					
	Insulin					
	Sugar					
	Insulin					
	Sugar					
	Insulin					

Weekly Meal Plan

Breakfast	Lunch	Dinner	Snacks	Sunday

Breakfast	Lunch	Dinner	Snacks	Monday

Breakfast	Lunch	Dinner	Snacks	Tuesday

Breakfast	Lunch	Dinner	Snacks	Wednesday

Breakfast	Lunch	Dinner	Snacks	Thursday

Breakfast	Lunch	Dinner	Snacks	Friday

Breakfast	Lunch	Dinner	Snacks	Saturday

Notes:

Food & Fitness Tracker

WEEK:_____

STARTING WEIGHT: _____

	CALORIE INTAKE		EXERCISE		
MON	BRKFST:		TYPE	TIME	CAL. BURNED
	LUNCH:				
	DINNER:				
	SNACKS:	BEVERAGES:			
	TOTAL CALORIE INTAKE:		**TOTAL CALORIES BURNED:**		
TUE	BRKFST:		TYPE	TIME	CAL. BURNED
	LUNCH:				
	DINNER:				
	SNACKS:	BEVERAGES:			
	TOTAL CALORIE INTAKE:		**TOTAL CALORIES BURNED:**		
WED	BRKFST:		TYPE	TIME	CAL. BURNED
	LUNCH:				
	DINNER:				
	SNACKS:	BEVERAGES:			
	TOTAL CALORIE INTAKE:		**TOTAL CALORIES BURNED:**		
THU	BRKFST:		TYPE	TIME	CAL. BURNED
	LUNCH:				
	DINNER:				
	SNACKS:	BEVERAGES:			
	TOTAL CALORIE INTAKE:		**TOTAL CALORIES BURNED:**		
FRI	BRKFST:		TYPE	TIME	CAL. BURNED
	LUNCH:				
	DINNER:				
	SNACKS:	BEVERAGES:			
	TOTAL CALORIE INTAKE:		**TOTAL CALORIES BURNED:**		
SAT	BRKFST:		TYPE	TIME	CAL. BURNED
	LUNCH:				
	DINNER:				
	SNACKS:	BEVERAGES:			
	TOTAL CALORIE INTAKE:		**TOTAL CALORIES BURNED:**		
SUN	BRKFST:		TYPE	TIME	CAL. BURNED
	LUNCH:				
	DINNER:				
	SNACKS:	BEVERAGES:			

ENDING WEIGHT: _____   Lost/Gained _____

Weekly Plans

Sunday

Monday

Tuesday

Wednesday

Thursday

Friday

Saturday

Date		AM	NOON	SUPPER	BEDTIME	WEIGHT
	Sugar					
	Insulin					
	Sugar					
	Insulin					
	Sugar					
	Insulin					
	Sugar					
	Insulin					
	Sugar					
	Insulin					
	Sugar					
	Insulin					
	Sugar					
	Insulin					

Weekly Meal Plan

| Breakfast | Lunch | Dinner | Snacks | Sunday |

| Breakfast | Lunch | Dinner | Snacks | Monday |

| Breakfast | Lunch | Dinner | Snacks | Tuesday |

| Breakfast | Lunch | Dinner | Snacks | Wednesday |

| Breakfast | Lunch | Dinner | Snacks | Thursday |

| Breakfast | Lunch | Dinner | Snacks | Friday |

| Breakfast | Lunch | Dinner | Snacks | Saturday |

Notes:

Food & Fitness Tracker

WEEK:_____

STARTING WEIGHT: _____

CALORIE INTAKE		EXERCISE		

MON
		TYPE	TIME	CAL. BURNED
BRKFST:				
LUNCH:				
DINNER:				
SNACKS:	BEVERAGES:			
TOTAL CALORIE INTAKE:		**TOTAL CALORIES BURNED:**		

TUE
		TYPE	TIME	CAL. BURNED
BRKFST:				
LUNCH:				
DINNER:				
SNACKS:	BEVERAGES:			
TOTAL CALORIE INTAKE:		**TOTAL CALORIES BURNED:**		

WED
		TYPE	TIME	CAL. BURNED
BRKFST:				
LUNCH:				
DINNER:				
SNACKS:	BEVERAGES:			
TOTAL CALORIE INTAKE:		**TOTAL CALORIES BURNED:**		

THU
		TYPE	TIME	CAL. BURNED
BRKFST:				
LUNCH:				
DINNER:				
SNACKS:	BEVERAGES:			
TOTAL CALORIE INTAKE:		**TOTAL CALORIES BURNED:**		

FRI
		TYPE	TIME	CAL. BURNED
BRKFST:				
LUNCH:				
DINNER:				
SNACKS:	BEVERAGES:			
TOTAL CALORIE INTAKE:		**TOTAL CALORIES BURNED:**		

SAT
		TYPE	TIME	CAL. BURNED
BRKFST:				
LUNCH:				
DINNER:				
SNACKS:	BEVERAGES:			
TOTAL CALORIE INTAKE:		**TOTAL CALORIES BURNED:**		

SUN
		TYPE	TIME	CAL. BURNED
BRKFST:				
LUNCH:				
DINNER:				
SNACKS:	BEVERAGES:			

ENDING WEIGHT: _____   Lost/Gained _____

Weekly Plans

	Sunday

	Monday

	Tuesday

	Wednesday

	Thursday

	Friday

	Saturday

Date		AM	NOON	SUPPER	BEDTIME	WEIGHT
	Sugar					
	Insulin					
	Sugar					
	Insulin					
	Sugar					
	Insulin					
	Sugar					
	Insulin					
	Sugar					
	Insulin					
	Sugar					
	Insulin					
	Sugar					
	Insulin					

Weekly Meal Plan

Breakfast	Lunch	Dinner	Snacks	Sunday

Breakfast	Lunch	Dinner	Snacks	Monday

Breakfast	Lunch	Dinner	Snacks	Tuesday

Breakfast	Lunch	Dinner	Snacks	Wednesday

Breakfast	Lunch	Dinner	Snacks	Thursday

Breakfast	Lunch	Dinner	Snacks	Friday

Breakfast	Lunch	Dinner	Snacks	Saturday

Notes:

Food & Fitness Tracker

CALORIE INTAKE		EXERCISE		
		TYPE	TIME	CAL. BURNED

MON
CALORIE INTAKE		EXERCISE		
BRKFST:		TYPE	TIME	CAL. BURNED
LUNCH:				
DINNER:				
SNACKS:	BEVERAGES:			
TOTAL CALORIE INTAKE:		**TOTAL CALORIES BURNED:**		

TUE
BRKFST:		TYPE	TIME	CAL. BURNED
LUNCH:				
DINNER:				
SNACKS:	BEVERAGES:			
TOTAL CALORIE INTAKE:		**TOTAL CALORIES BURNED:**		

WED
BRKFST:		TYPE	TIME	CAL. BURNED
LUNCH:				
DINNER:				
SNACKS:	BEVERAGES:			
TOTAL CALORIE INTAKE:		**TOTAL CALORIES BURNED:**		

THU
BRKFST:		TYPE	TIME	CAL. BURNED
LUNCH:				
DINNER:				
SNACKS:	BEVERAGES:			
TOTAL CALORIE INTAKE:		**TOTAL CALORIES BURNED:**		

FRI
BRKFST:		TYPE	TIME	CAL. BURNED
LUNCH:				
DINNER:				
SNACKS:	BEVERAGES:			
TOTAL CALORIE INTAKE:		**TOTAL CALORIES BURNED:**		

SAT
BRKFST:		TYPE	TIME	CAL. BURNED
LUNCH:				
DINNER:				
SNACKS:	BEVERAGES:			
TOTAL CALORIE INTAKE:		**TOTAL CALORIES BURNED:**		

SUN
BRKFST:		TYPE	TIME	CAL. BURNED
LUNCH:				
DINNER:				
SNACKS:	BEVERAGES:			

ENDING WEIGHT: _____   Lost/Gained _____

Weekly Plans

	Sunday

	Monday

	Tuesday

	Wednesday

	Thursday

	Friday

	Saturday

Date		AM	NOON	SUPPER	BEDTIME	WEIGHT
	Sugar					
	Insulin					
	Sugar					
	Insulin					
	Sugar					
	Insulin					
	Sugar					
	Insulin					
	Sugar					
	Insulin					
	Sugar					
	Insulin					
	Sugar					
	Insulin					

Weekly Meal Plan

Breakfast	Lunch	Dinner	Snacks	
				Sunday

Breakfast	Lunch	Dinner	Snacks	
				Monday

Breakfast	Lunch	Dinner	Snacks	
				Tuesday

Breakfast	Lunch	Dinner	Snacks	
				Wednesday

Breakfast	Lunch	Dinner	Snacks	
				Thursday

Breakfast	Lunch	Dinner	Snacks	
				Friday

Breakfast	Lunch	Dinner	Snacks	
				Saturday

Notes:

Food & Fitness Tracker

WEEK:_____

STARTING WEIGHT: _____

CALORIE INTAKE		EXERCISE		

MON
CALORIE INTAKE	EXERCISE			
BRKFST:		TYPE	TIME	CAL. BURNED
LUNCH:				
DINNER:				
SNACKS:	BEVERAGES:			
TOTAL CALORIE INTAKE:		TOTAL CALORIES BURNED:		

TUE
BRKFST:		TYPE	TIME	CAL. BURNED
LUNCH:				
DINNER:				
SNACKS:	BEVERAGES:			
TOTAL CALORIE INTAKE:		TOTAL CALORIES BURNED:		

WED
BRKFST:		TYPE	TIME	CAL. BURNED
LUNCH:				
DINNER:				
SNACKS:	BEVERAGES:			
TOTAL CALORIE INTAKE:		TOTAL CALORIES BURNED:		

THU
BRKFST:		TYPE	TIME	CAL. BURNED
LUNCH:				
DINNER:				
SNACKS:	BEVERAGES:			
TOTAL CALORIE INTAKE:		TOTAL CALORIES BURNED:		

FRI
BRKFST:		TYPE	TIME	CAL. BURNED
LUNCH:				
DINNER:				
SNACKS:	BEVERAGES:			
TOTAL CALORIE INTAKE:		TOTAL CALORIES BURNED:		

SAT
BRKFST:		TYPE	TIME	CAL. BURNED
LUNCH:				
DINNER:				
SNACKS:	BEVERAGES:			
TOTAL CALORIE INTAKE:		TOTAL CALORIES BURNED:		

SUN
BRKFST:		TYPE	TIME	CAL. BURNED
LUNCH:				
DINNER:				
SNACKS:	BEVERAGES:			

ENDING WEIGHT: _____   Lost/Gained _____

Weekly Plans

Sunday

Monday

Tuesday

Wednesday

Thursday

Friday

Saturday

Date		AM	NOON	SUPPER	BEDTIME	WEIGHT
	Sugar					
	Insulin					
	Sugar					
	Insulin					
	Sugar					
	Insulin					
	Sugar					
	Insulin					
	Sugar					
	Insulin					
	Sugar					
	Insulin					
	Sugar					
	Insulin					

Weekly Meal Plan

Breakfast	Lunch	Dinner	Snacks	
				Sunday

Breakfast	Lunch	Dinner	Snacks	
				Monday

Breakfast	Lunch	Dinner	Snacks	
				Tuesday

Breakfast	Lunch	Dinner	Snacks	
				Wednesday

Breakfast	Lunch	Dinner	Snacks	
				Thursday

Breakfast	Lunch	Dinner	Snacks	
				Friday

Breakfast	Lunch	Dinner	Snacks	
				Saturday

Notes:

Food & Fitness Tracker

WEEK:_____

STARTING WEIGHT:_____

	CALORIE INTAKE		EXERCISE		
MON	BRKFST:		TYPE	TIME	CAL. BURNED
	LUNCH:				
	DINNER:				
	SNACKS:	BEVERAGES:			
	TOTAL CALORIE INTAKE:		**TOTAL CALORIES BURNED:**		
TUE	BRKFST:		TYPE	TIME	CAL. BURNED
	LUNCH:				
	DINNER:				
	SNACKS:	BEVERAGES:			
	TOTAL CALORIE INTAKE:		**TOTAL CALORIES BURNED:**		
WED	BRKFST:		TYPE	TIME	CAL. BURNED
	LUNCH:				
	DINNER:				
	SNACKS:	BEVERAGES:			
	TOTAL CALORIE INTAKE:		**TOTAL CALORIES BURNED:**		
THU	BRKFST:		TYPE	TIME	CAL. BURNED
	LUNCH:				
	DINNER:				
	SNACKS:	BEVERAGES:			
	TOTAL CALORIE INTAKE:		**TOTAL CALORIES BURNED:**		
FRI	BRKFST:		TYPE	TIME	CAL. BURNED
	LUNCH:				
	DINNER:				
	SNACKS:	BEVERAGES:			
	TOTAL CALORIE INTAKE:		**TOTAL CALORIES BURNED:**		
SAT	BRKFST:		TYPE	TIME	CAL. BURNED
	LUNCH:				
	DINNER:				
	SNACKS:	BEVERAGES:			
	TOTAL CALORIE INTAKE:		**TOTAL CALORIES BURNED:**		
SUN	BRKFST:		TYPE	TIME	CAL. BURNED
	LUNCH:				
	DINNER:				
	SNACKS:	BEVERAGES:			

ENDING WEIGHT: _____   Lost/Gained _____

Weekly Plans

Sunday

Monday

Tuesday

Wednesday

Thursday

Friday

Saturday

Date		AM	NOON	SUPPER	BEDTIME	WEIGHT
	Sugar					
	Insulin					
	Sugar					
	Insulin					
	Sugar					
	Insulin					
	Sugar					
	Insulin					
	Sugar					
	Insulin					
	Sugar					
	Insulin					
	Sugar					
	Insulin					

Weekly Meal Plan

| Breakfast | Lunch | Dinner | Snacks | Sunday |

| Breakfast | Lunch | Dinner | Snacks | Monday |

| Breakfast | Lunch | Dinner | Snacks | Tuesday |

| Breakfast | Lunch | Dinner | Snacks | Wednesday |

| Breakfast | Lunch | Dinner | Snacks | Thursday |

| Breakfast | Lunch | Dinner | Snacks | Friday |

| Breakfast | Lunch | Dinner | Snacks | Saturday |

Notes:

Food & Fitness Tracker

WEEK:_____

STARTING WEIGHT:_____

	CALORIE INTAKE		EXERCISE		
MON	BRKFST:		TYPE	TIME	CAL. BURNED
	LUNCH:				
	DINNER:				
	SNACKS:	BEVERAGES:			
	TOTAL CALORIE INTAKE:		**TOTAL CALORIES BURNED:**		
TUE	BRKFST:		TYPE	TIME	CAL. BURNED
	LUNCH:				
	DINNER:				
	SNACKS:	BEVERAGES:			
	TOTAL CALORIE INTAKE:		**TOTAL CALORIES BURNED:**		
WED	BRKFST:		TYPE	TIME	CAL. BURNED
	LUNCH:				
	DINNER:				
	SNACKS:	BEVERAGES:			
	TOTAL CALORIE INTAKE:		**TOTAL CALORIES BURNED:**		
THU	BRKFST:		TYPE	TIME	CAL. BURNED
	LUNCH:				
	DINNER:				
	SNACKS:	BEVERAGES:			
	TOTAL CALORIE INTAKE:		**TOTAL CALORIES BURNED:**		
FRI	BRKFST:		TYPE	TIME	CAL. BURNED
	LUNCH:				
	DINNER:				
	SNACKS:	BEVERAGES:			
	TOTAL CALORIE INTAKE:		**TOTAL CALORIES BURNED:**		
SAT	BRKFST:		TYPE	TIME	CAL. BURNED
	LUNCH:				
	DINNER:				
	SNACKS:	BEVERAGES:			
	TOTAL CALORIE INTAKE:		**TOTAL CALORIES BURNED:**		
SUN	BRKFST:		TYPE	TIME	CAL. BURNED
	LUNCH:				
	DINNER:				
	SNACKS:	BEVERAGES:			

ENDING WEIGHT: _____   Lost/Gained _____

Weekly Plans

Sunday

Monday

Tuesday

Wednesday

Thursday

Friday

Saturday

Date		AM	NOON	SUPPER	BEDTIME	WEIGHT
	Sugar					
	Insulin					
	Sugar					
	Insulin					
	Sugar					
	Insulin					
	Sugar					
	Insulin					
	Sugar					
	Insulin					
	Sugar					
	Insulin					
	Sugar					
	Insulin					

Weekly Meal Plan

Breakfast	Lunch	Dinner	Snacks	Sunday

Breakfast	Lunch	Dinner	Snacks	Monday

Breakfast	Lunch	Dinner	Snacks	Tuesday

Breakfast	Lunch	Dinner	Snacks	Wednesday

Breakfast	Lunch	Dinner	Snacks	Thursday

Breakfast	Lunch	Dinner	Snacks	Friday

Breakfast	Lunch	Dinner	Snacks	Saturday

Notes:

Food & Fitness Tracker

CALORIE INTAKE		EXERCISE		
MON				
BRKFST:		TYPE	TIME	CAL. BURNED
LUNCH:				
DINNER:				
SNACKS:	BEVERAGES:			
TOTAL CALORIE INTAKE:		**TOTAL CALORIES BURNED:**		
TUE				
BRKFST:		TYPE	TIME	CAL. BURNED
LUNCH:				
DINNER:				
SNACKS:	BEVERAGES:			
TOTAL CALORIE INTAKE:		**TOTAL CALORIES BURNED:**		
WED				
BRKFST:		TYPE	TIME	CAL. BURNED
LUNCH:				
DINNER:				
SNACKS:	BEVERAGES:			
TOTAL CALORIE INTAKE:		**TOTAL CALORIES BURNED:**		
THU				
BRKFST:		TYPE	TIME	CAL. BURNED
LUNCH:				
DINNER:				
SNACKS:	BEVERAGES:			
TOTAL CALORIE INTAKE:		**TOTAL CALORIES BURNED:**		
FRI				
BRKFST:		TYPE	TIME	CAL. BURNED
LUNCH:				
DINNER:				
SNACKS:	BEVERAGES:			
TOTAL CALORIE INTAKE:		**TOTAL CALORIES BURNED:**		
SAT				
BRKFST:		TYPE	TIME	CAL. BURNED
LUNCH:				
DINNER:				
SNACKS:	BEVERAGES:			
TOTAL CALORIE INTAKE:		**TOTAL CALORIES BURNED:**		
SUN				
BRKFST:		TYPE	TIME	CAL. BURNED
LUNCH:				
DINNER:				
SNACKS:	BEVERAGES:			

ENDING WEIGHT: _____   Lost/Gained _____

Weekly Plans

Sunday

Monday

Tuesday

Wednesday

Thursday

Friday

Saturday

Date		AM	NOON	SUPPER	BEDTIME	WEIGHT
	Sugar					
	Insulin					
	Sugar					
	Insulin					
	Sugar					
	Insulin					
	Sugar					
	Insulin					
	Sugar					
	Insulin					
	Sugar					
	Insulin					
	Sugar					
	Insulin					

Weekly Meal Plan

Breakfast	Lunch	Dinner	Snacks	
				Sunday

Breakfast	Lunch	Dinner	Snacks	
				Monday

Breakfast	Lunch	Dinner	Snacks	
				Tuesday

Breakfast	Lunch	Dinner	Snacks	
				Wednesday

Breakfast	Lunch	Dinner	Snacks	
				Thursday

Breakfast	Lunch	Dinner	Snacks	
				Friday

Breakfast	Lunch	Dinner	Snacks	
				Saturday

Notes:

Food & Fitness Tracker

WEEK: _____

STARTING WEIGHT: _____

	CALORIE INTAKE		EXERCISE		
MON	BRKFST:		TYPE	TIME	CAL. BURNED
	LUNCH:				
	DINNER:				
	SNACKS:	BEVERAGES:			
	TOTAL CALORIE INTAKE:		**TOTAL CALORIES BURNED:**		
TUE	BRKFST:		TYPE	TIME	CAL. BURNED
	LUNCH:				
	DINNER:				
	SNACKS:	BEVERAGES:			
	TOTAL CALORIE INTAKE:		**TOTAL CALORIES BURNED:**		
WED	BRKFST:		TYPE	TIME	CAL. BURNED
	LUNCH:				
	DINNER:				
	SNACKS:	BEVERAGES:			
	TOTAL CALORIE INTAKE:		**TOTAL CALORIES BURNED:**		
THU	BRKFST:		TYPE	TIME	CAL. BURNED
	LUNCH:				
	DINNER:				
	SNACKS:	BEVERAGES:			
	TOTAL CALORIE INTAKE:		**TOTAL CALORIES BURNED:**		
FRI	BRKFST:		TYPE	TIME	CAL. BURNED
	LUNCH:				
	DINNER:				
	SNACKS:	BEVERAGES:			
	TOTAL CALORIE INTAKE:		**TOTAL CALORIES BURNED:**		
SAT	BRKFST:		TYPE	TIME	CAL. BURNED
	LUNCH:				
	DINNER:				
	SNACKS:	BEVERAGES:			
	TOTAL CALORIE INTAKE:		**TOTAL CALORIES BURNED:**		
SUN	BRKFST:		TYPE	TIME	CAL. BURNED
	LUNCH:				
	DINNER:				
	SNACKS:	BEVERAGES:			

ENDING WEIGHT: _____

Lost/Gained _____

Weekly Plans

Sunday

Monday

Tuesday

Wednesday

Thursday

Friday

Saturday

Date		AM	NOON	SUPPER	BEDTIME	WEIGHT
	Sugar					
	Insulin					
	Sugar					
	Insulin					
	Sugar					
	Insulin					
	Sugar					
	Insulin					
	Sugar					
	Insulin					
	Sugar					
	Insulin					
	Sugar					
	Insulin					

Weekly Meal Plan

Breakfast	Lunch	Dinner	Snacks	Sunday

Breakfast	Lunch	Dinner	Snacks	Monday

Breakfast	Lunch	Dinner	Snacks	Tuesday

Breakfast	Lunch	Dinner	Snacks	Wednesday

Breakfast	Lunch	Dinner	Snacks	Thursday

Breakfast	Lunch	Dinner	Snacks	Friday

Breakfast	Lunch	Dinner	Snacks	Saturday

Notes:

Food & Fitness Tracker

WEEK: _____

STARTING WEIGHT: _____

	CALORIE INTAKE			EXERCISE		
MON	BRKFST:			TYPE	TIME	CAL. BURNED
	LUNCH:					
	DINNER:					
	SNACKS:	BEVERAGES:				
	TOTAL CALORIE INTAKE:			**TOTAL CALORIES BURNED:**		
TUE	BRKFST:			TYPE	TIME	CAL. BURNED
	LUNCH:					
	DINNER:					
	SNACKS:	BEVERAGES:				
	TOTAL CALORIE INTAKE:			**TOTAL CALORIES BURNED:**		
WED	BRKFST:			TYPE	TIME	CAL. BURNED
	LUNCH:					
	DINNER:					
	SNACKS:	BEVERAGES:				
	TOTAL CALORIE INTAKE:			**TOTAL CALORIES BURNED:**		
THU	BRKFST:			TYPE	TIME	CAL. BURNED
	LUNCH:					
	DINNER:					
	SNACKS:	BEVERAGES:				
	TOTAL CALORIE INTAKE:			**TOTAL CALORIES BURNED:**		
FRI	BRKFST:			TYPE	TIME	CAL. BURNED
	LUNCH:					
	DINNER:					
	SNACKS:	BEVERAGES:				
	TOTAL CALORIE INTAKE:			**TOTAL CALORIES BURNED:**		
SAT	BRKFST:			TYPE	TIME	CAL. BURNED
	LUNCH:					
	DINNER:					
	SNACKS:	BEVERAGES:				
	TOTAL CALORIE INTAKE:			**TOTAL CALORIES BURNED:**		
SUN	BRKFST:			TYPE	TIME	CAL. BURNED
	LUNCH:					
	DINNER:					
	SNACKS:	BEVERAGES:				

ENDING WEIGHT: _____   Lost/Gained _____

Weekly Plans

Sunday

Monday

Tuesday

Wednesday

Thursday

Friday

Saturday

Date		AM	NOON	SUPPER	BEDTIME	WEIGHT
	Sugar					
	Insulin					
	Sugar					
	Insulin					
	Sugar					
	Insulin					
	Sugar					
	Insulin					
	Sugar					
	Insulin					
	Sugar					
	Insulin					
	Sugar					
	Insulin					

Weekly Meal Plan

Breakfast	Lunch	Dinner	Snacks	Sunday

Breakfast	Lunch	Dinner	Snacks	Monday

Breakfast	Lunch	Dinner	Snacks	Tuesday

Breakfast	Lunch	Dinner	Snacks	Wednesday

Breakfast	Lunch	Dinner	Snacks	Thursday

Breakfast	Lunch	Dinner	Snacks	Friday

Breakfast	Lunch	Dinner	Snacks	Saturday

Notes:

Food & Fitness Tracker

WEEK:_____

STARTING WEIGHT: _____

	CALORIE INTAKE		EXERCISE		
MON	BRKFST:		TYPE	TIME	CAL. BURNED
	LUNCH:				
	DINNER:				
	SNACKS:	BEVERAGES:			
	TOTAL CALORIE INTAKE:		**TOTAL CALORIES BURNED:**		
TUE	BRKFST:		TYPE	TIME	CAL. BURNED
	LUNCH:				
	DINNER:				
	SNACKS:	BEVERAGES:			
	TOTAL CALORIE INTAKE:		**TOTAL CALORIES BURNED:**		
WED	BRKFST:		TYPE	TIME	CAL. BURNED
	LUNCH:				
	DINNER:				
	SNACKS:	BEVERAGES:			
	TOTAL CALORIE INTAKE:		**TOTAL CALORIES BURNED:**		
THU	BRKFST:		TYPE	TIME	CAL. BURNED
	LUNCH:				
	DINNER:				
	SNACKS:	BEVERAGES:			
	TOTAL CALORIE INTAKE:		**TOTAL CALORIES BURNED:**		
FRI	BRKFST:		TYPE	TIME	CAL. BURNED
	LUNCH:				
	DINNER:				
	SNACKS:	BEVERAGES:			
	TOTAL CALORIE INTAKE:		**TOTAL CALORIES BURNED:**		
SAT	BRKFST:		TYPE	TIME	CAL. BURNED
	LUNCH:				
	DINNER:				
	SNACKS:	BEVERAGES:			
	TOTAL CALORIE INTAKE:		**TOTAL CALORIES BURNED:**		
SUN	BRKFST:		TYPE	TIME	CAL. BURNED
	LUNCH:				
	DINNER:				
	SNACKS:	BEVERAGES:			

ENDING WEIGHT: _____   Lost/Gained _____

Weekly Plans

	Sunday

	Monday

	Tuesday

	Wednesday

	Thursday

	Friday

	Saturday

Date		AM	NOON	SUPPER	BEDTIME	WEIGHT
	Sugar					
	Insulin					
	Sugar					
	Insulin					
	Sugar					
	Insulin					
	Sugar					
	Insulin					
	Sugar					
	Insulin					
	Sugar					
	Insulin					
	Sugar					
	Insulin					

Weekly Meal Plan

Breakfast	Lunch	Dinner	Snacks	Sunday

Breakfast	Lunch	Dinner	Snacks	Monday

Breakfast	Lunch	Dinner	Snacks	Tuesday

Breakfast	Lunch	Dinner	Snacks	Wednesday

Breakfast	Lunch	Dinner	Snacks	Thursday

Breakfast	Lunch	Dinner	Snacks	Friday

Breakfast	Lunch	Dinner	Snacks	Saturday

Notes:

Food & Fitness Tracker

WEEK:_____

STARTING WEIGHT:_____

CALORIE INTAKE		EXERCISE		

MON

BRKFST:		TYPE	TIME	CAL. BURNED
LUNCH:				
DINNER:				
SNACKS:	BEVERAGES:			
TOTAL CALORIE INTAKE:		**TOTAL CALORIES BURNED:**		

TUE

BRKFST:		TYPE	TIME	CAL. BURNED
LUNCH:				
DINNER:				
SNACKS:	BEVERAGES:			
TOTAL CALORIE INTAKE:		**TOTAL CALORIES BURNED:**		

WED

BRKFST:		TYPE	TIME	CAL. BURNED
LUNCH:				
DINNER:				
SNACKS:	BEVERAGES:			
TOTAL CALORIE INTAKE:		**TOTAL CALORIES BURNED:**		

THU

BRKFST:		TYPE	TIME	CAL. BURNED
LUNCH:				
DINNER:				
SNACKS:	BEVERAGES:			
TOTAL CALORIE INTAKE:		**TOTAL CALORIES BURNED:**		

FRI

BRKFST:		TYPE	TIME	CAL. BURNED
LUNCH:				
DINNER:				
SNACKS:	BEVERAGES:			
TOTAL CALORIE INTAKE:		**TOTAL CALORIES BURNED:**		

SAT

BRKFST:		TYPE	TIME	CAL. BURNED
LUNCH:				
DINNER:				
SNACKS:	BEVERAGES:			
TOTAL CALORIE INTAKE:		**TOTAL CALORIES BURNED:**		

SUN

BRKFST:		TYPE	TIME	CAL. BURNED
LUNCH:				
DINNER:				
SNACKS:	BEVERAGES:			

ENDING WEIGHT: _____   Lost/Gained _____

Weekly Plans

	Sunday

	Monday

	Tuesday

	Wednesday

	Thursday

	Friday

	Saturday

Date		AM	NOON	SUPPER	BEDTIME	WEIGHT
	Sugar					
	Insulin					
	Sugar					
	Insulin					
	Sugar					
	Insulin					
	Sugar					
	Insulin					
	Sugar					
	Insulin					
	Sugar					
	Insulin					
	Sugar					
	Insulin					

Notes to myself or Goals I need to set up so that I will not lose a leg or toes or fingers.

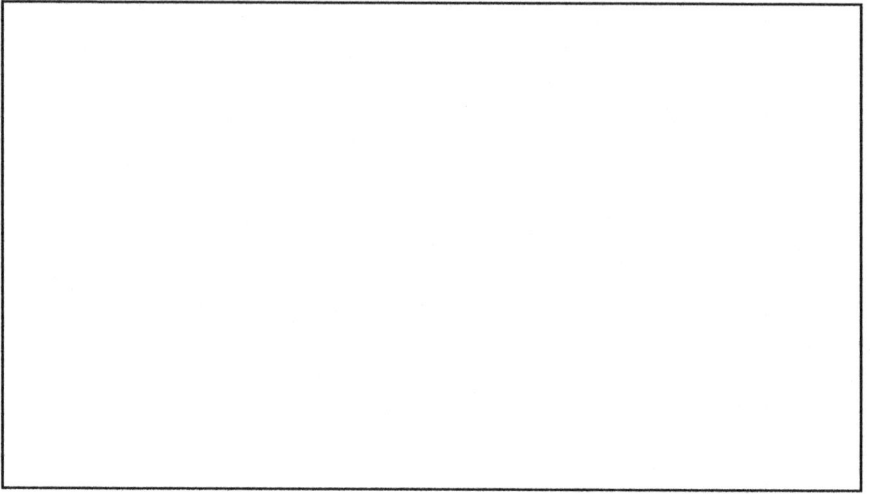

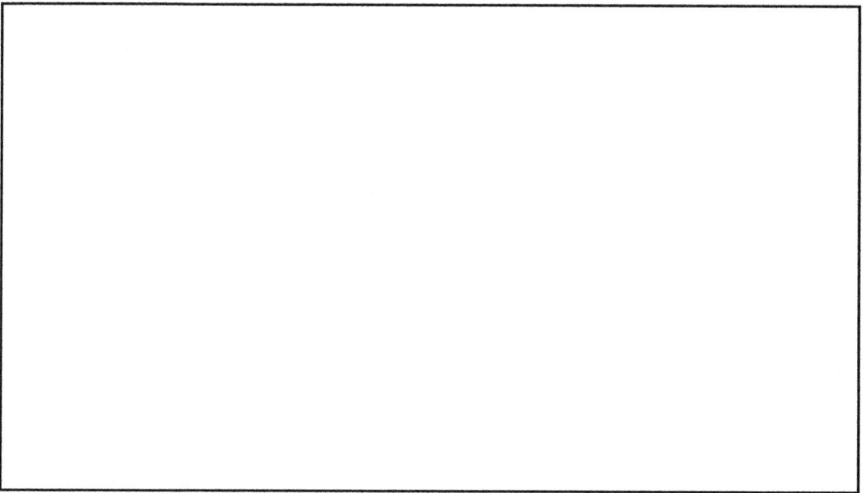

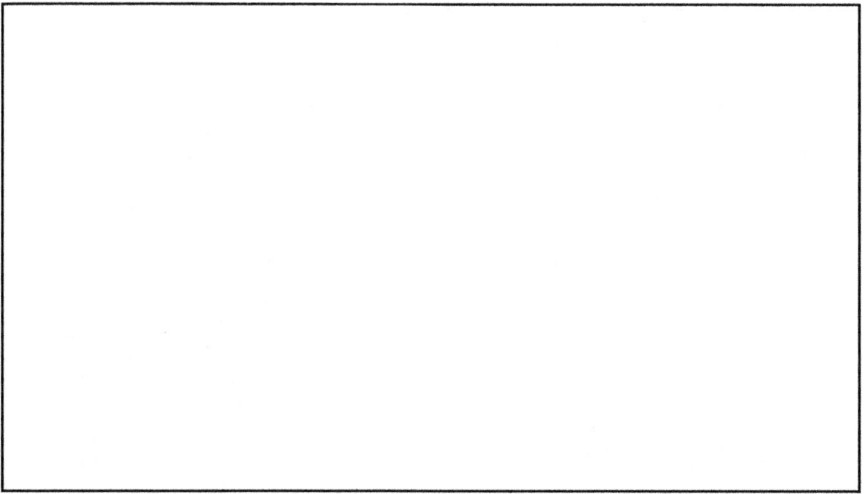

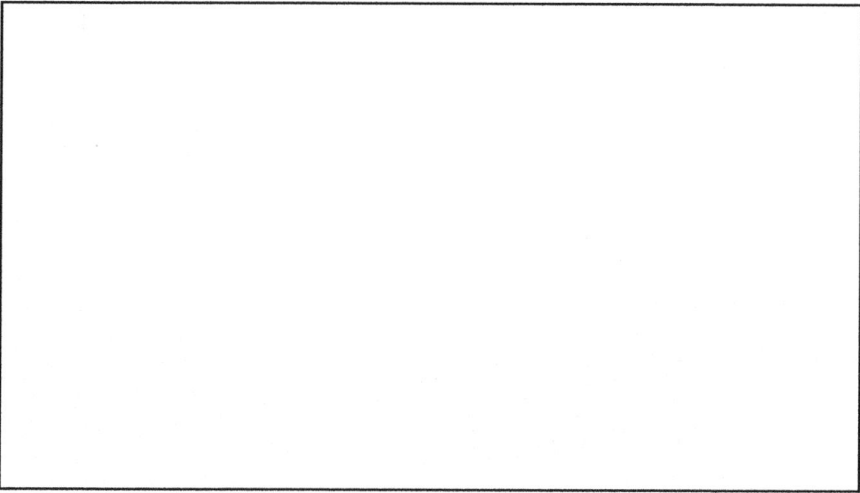

Made in the USA
Las Vegas, NV
22 February 2022